OVERCOMING JEALOUSY & INSECURITY IN RELATIONSHIP

Breaking Free From Anxiety, Master your Emotions, Learn to Trust and Revive your Self-Worth

Andrew Wiseman

INTRODUCTION

CHAPTER ONE

HOW TO DEAL WITH JEALOUSY

What to Do:

CHAPTER TWO

OPEN MIND

FOLLOW IT BACK TO ITS SOURCE:

VOICE YOUR INTERESTS:

CHAPTER THREE

CONSIDER THE WHOLE PICTURE

CAUSES WEAKNESS IN A RELATIONSHIP

CHAPTER FOUR

FIXING LOW SELF-ESTEEM IN A RELATIONSHIP

CHAPTER FIVE

INTERACTING WITH YOUR PARTNER

INTRODUCTION

To show how this inward foe takes care of our negative feelings around jealousy, we'll take a gander at two kinds of desire: heartfelt envy and serious desire. While these two types of jealousy regularly cross-over, considering them independently can assist us with bettering envious feelings might be influencing various parts of our lives and how we can best arrangement with desire.

Romantic jealousy: It's an essential reality that connections go smoother when individuals don't get excessively desirous. The more we can take a few to get back some composure on our feelings of jealousy and figure out them separate from our accomplice, the good we will be. Keep in mind, our jealousy frequently comes from uncertainty in ourselves – a feeling like we are bound to be misled, harmed or dismissed. Except if we manage this inclination in ourselves, we are probably going to succumb to sensations of desire, doubt or weakness in any relationship, regardless the conditions.

These negative feelings about ourselves begin from early encounters in our lives. We frequently take on feelings our folks or significant guardians had toward us or toward themselves. We then, at that point, unknowingly, replay, reproduce or respond to old, natural elements in our present connections. For instance, in the event that we felt cast to the side as children, we may handily see our accomplice as overlooking us. We may pick an accomplice who's more subtle or even participate in practices that would drive our accomplice away.

The degree to which we took on self-basic mentalities as kids frequently shapes how much our basic inward voice will influence us in our grown-up lives, particularly in our connections. However, regardless our extraordinary encounters might be, we as a whole have this inward pundit somewhat. The vast majority of us can identify with hauling around an inclination that we will not be picked. How much we accept this dread influences how compromised we will feel in a relationship.

These jealousy inclination can emerge anytime in a relationship, from a first date to the twentieth year of a marriage. While trying to secure ourselves, we may pay attention to our inward pundit and pull back from being near our accomplice. However, in an extreme difficult situation, we likewise will in general feel more envious when we've withdrawn from seeking after what we need. In the event that we know in some way or another we're not focusing on our relationship or effectively pursuing our objective of being adoring or close, we will in general feel more unreliable and more envious. That is the reason it's considerably more fundamental to figure out how to manage envy and not to aimlessly follow up on envious sentiments by driving our accomplice further away.

Competitive Jealousy: While it might feel silly or unreasonable, it is totally normal to need what others have and to feel serious. Notwithstanding, how we utilize these feelings is vital to our degree of fulfillment and bliss. In the event that we utilize these feelings to serve our inward pundit, to destroy ourselves or others, that is unmistakably a ruinous example with discouraging impacts. Notwithstanding, on the off chance that we don't allow these feelings to fall under the control of our basic internal voice, we can really utilize them to recognize what we need, to be more objective coordinated or even to feel more tolerating of ourselves and what influences us.

It's alright, even solid, to permit ourselves to have a serious idea. It can feel great when we just let ourselves have the flitting feeling without judgment or an arrangement for activity. In any case, on the off chance that we ruminate or contort this idea into an analysis of ourselves or an assault on someone else, we end up getting injured. In the event that we wind up having an overcompensation or feeling frequented by our sensations of jealousy, we can complete a few things.

Know about what gets set off. Consider the particular occasions that cause you to feel worked up. Is it a companion who's having monetary achievement? An ex who's dating another person? A colleague who expresses her genuine thoughts in gatherings?

Ask yourself what basic inward voices come up. What kinds of contemplations do these desirous sentiments sparkle? Is it accurate to say that you are utilizing these sensations of envy to put yourself down? Do they cause you to feel unimportant, unable, and fruitless and so on? Is there an example or topic to these musings that feels recognizable?

Consider the more profound ramifications and beginnings of these contemplations: Do you feel a specific strain to accomplish something specific? Is there something you believe you should be? What might getting this thing mean about you? Does this interface with your past?

Whenever we've asked ourselves these inquiries, we can see how these sentiments may have more to do with irritating issues inside us than with our present life or the individual our envy is aimed at. We can have more empathy for ourselves and attempt to suspend the decisions that lead us to feel uncertain.

CHAPTER ONE

HOW TO DEAL WITH JEALOUSY

What to Do:

Quiet down and stay defenseless:

Regardless of how jealous we believe, we can discover approaches to return to ourselves and relax. We can do this by first, tolerating our feelings with empathy. Recall that regardless of how solid we feel, our feelings will in general pass in waves, first structure, then, at that point dying down. It's feasible to acknowledge constantly our desire without following up on it. We can learn instruments to quiet ourselves down prior to responding, for instance, by going for a stroll or a progression of full breaths. It's significantly simpler to quiet down in this manner when we won't endure or enjoy the furious expressions of our internal pundit, so learning steps to challenge it is fundamental. At the point when we do, we can tolerate upping for ourselves and individuals we care for and stay powerless and open by the way we relate.

Try not to carry on:

 Our basic inward voice will in general encourage us to make moves that can hurt us over the long run. When it twisting us into a condition of jealousy, it might advise us to surrender or quit following what we need. It might lead us to self-harm, explode at or rebuff somebody we regard. In case we're seeing someone, may advise us to ice or lash out at our accomplice. At the point when we do this, everything we do is make the powerful we're apprehensive about. We may offend and sabotage our accomplices' for us and work up their own sensations of doubt and dread. We may coincidentally urge them to turn out to be more stopped, less open about their sentiments, musings and activities, which then, at that point adds to our sensations of doubt and desire.

Look for our own conviction that all is good:

Everything thing we can manage is center around feeling solid and secure in ourselves. We need to accomplish the work to overcome our internal pundit and accept that we are OK, even all alone. We needn't bother with one explicit individual's affection to accept we're loveable. People are brimming with imperfections and limits, and nobody can give us what we need 100% of the time. This is the reason practice self-empathy and figure out how to face our own internal pundit. This doesn't mean closing individuals out or stopping ourselves from what we need. It really implies accepting our lives sincere, while accepting that we're sufficiently able to fall flat or lose. Regardless, we can deal with the feelings that emerge.

Stay competitive – A many individuals disapprove of contending, however the thing we're discussing here isn't an objective of being the awesome, an individual objective of being at our best. That implies feeling such as ourselves and accepting the characteristics that will serve us in seeking after what we need. Maybe than allowing the green beast to transform us into beasts, we can permit ourselves to feel enlivened, to associate with who we need to be and make moves that carry us nearer to that. Assuming we need the admiration of people around us, we must be careful and obliging in our connections. Assuming we need to feel the predictable love of our accomplice, we should focus on participating in cherishing acts every single day. In the event that we keep a craving to act with honesty and pursue our objectives, we win the main fight we will confront, the battle to acknowledge and turn into our actual selves - separate from any other person.

Talk about it:

When something like desire is assuming control over, track down the opportune individual to converse with and a sound method to communicate what we feel. Individuals who support a positive side of us and who assist with preventing us from ruminating or sinking further into our distresses are the sort of companions we need to converse with about our desire. We as a whole have companions who get excessively stirred up when we raise certain subjects, and these may not be the dearest companions to search out when we ourselves are feeling set off and provoked up. We should attempt to discover individuals who will uphold us keeping focused and being the sort of people we need to be. Venting to these companions is fine as long as it's a question of letting out our silly contemplations and sentiments, while recognizing that they're misrepresented and unreasonable. This interaction works just when it diminishes us of the inclination and permits us to continue on and make sensible moves. In case we're enduring with sensations of desire, it's additionally extremely astute to look for the assistance of an advisor. This can help us figure out our feelings and understand them, while acting in better, versatile ways.

CHAPTER TWO
OPEN MIND

In a relationship, keep up with open, genuine correspondence with our accomplice. On the off chance that we desire to have their trust and for them to have our own, we need to pay attention to what they say without developing protective or racing to judgment. This open line of correspondence isn't tied in with emptying our uncertainties on our accomplice, however all things being equal, permitting ourselves to be benevolent and associated, in any event, when we feel shaky or desirous. This normally assists our band together with doing likewise.

Doubtlessly, that it takes a specific degree of enthusiastic development to manage the numerous sentiments around desire. It takes an ability to challenge our basic inward voice and every one of the frailties it creates. It likewise makes determination to stride back and oppose following up on our rash, desirous responses. Nonetheless, when we cultivate this force in ourselves, we understand we are significantly more grounded than we might suspect. By figuring out how to manage desire, we become safer in ourselves and in our connections.

Jealousy has a terrible standing. It's normal to hear good natured individuals make statements like, "Don't be envious" or "Envy annihilates connections." Yet what makes this feeling so awful?

While its normal connected to close connections, jealousy can come up at whatever point you're stressed over losing any person or thing imperative to you. This is not quite the same as jealousy, which includes needing something that has a place with another person.

Desire can prompt sensations of outrage, hatred, or bitterness. Yet, it can frequently scold you about yourself and your requirements.

Here's a gander at some approaches to adapt to desire and look at what's at the foundation of your sentiments.

FOLLOW IT BACK TO ITS SOURCE:

Analyzing your envious sentiments can give you knowledge on where they come from:

Your sister's new relationship causes desire since you haven't had a lot of karma dating and stress you'll never track down the perfect individual.

Your collaborator's advancement causes you to feel envious in light of the fact that you trust you're not sufficient at your responsibility to get an advancement yourself.

At the point when your accomplice begins investing a great deal of energy with another companion, you feel envious on the grounds that that was the primary sign you saw when a past accomplice cheated.

Regardless of whether your envy comes from frailty, dread, or past relationship designs, find out about the causes can help you sort out some way to defy it.

Perhaps you have an open discussion with your chief about refocusing for advancement, make plans to attempt an alternate way to deal with dating, or converse with your accomplice about your sentiments.

VOICE YOUR INTERESTS:

In case your accomplice's activities (or another person's activities toward your accomplice) trigger desirous sentiments, carry this up with your accomplice quickly.

Your accomplice might not have seen the conduct, or they might not have acknowledged how you felt about it. Utilize the chance to talk over any relationship limits you should return to, or examine approaches to keep your relationship solid. On the off chance that you trust your accomplice yet have questions in view of past relationship encounters, have a go at tracking down a couple of ways you both can assist with advancing the circumstance. In the event that you feel anxious about referencing envious sentiments, attempt to recall that they're absolutely ordinary. Your accomplice may even have had some envious sensations of their own eventually.

Converse with a confided in partner:

Desire can now and again give you a marginally twisted feeling of the real world. You may contemplate whether that nonverbal being a tease you swear you saw really occurred. At times, voicing these worries to an outsider can make the circumstance less terrifying and help you acquire some viewpoint.

Put an alternate twist on jealousy:

Envy can be an intricate, compelling feeling, and you probably won't feel excellent when you're managing it. However, rather than considering it something negative, have a go at viewing at it as an accommodating wellspring of data.

CHAPTER THREE

CONSIDER THE WHOLE PICTURE

Jealousy some of the time creates because of an incomplete picture. As such, you may be looking at yourself and your own accomplishments and qualities to a romanticized or deficient perspective on another person. In any case, you never genuinely realize what somebody's going through, particularly when you're simply taking a gander at web-based media.

Your school companion with the Facebook photographs of her and her better half out in a knoll, looking so lighthearted and cheerful? As far as you might be aware, they contended way out there and they're breaking out in a cold sweat under all that coordinating with plaid.

Practice appreciation for what you have:

A little appreciation can go far. It can diminish sensations of desire, yet in addition calm pressure.

You probably won't have all that you need. A large portion of us don't. Be that as it may, you likely have basically some of what you need. Possibly you even have some beneficial things in your day to day existence you didn't anticipate.

This can help whether you're peering toward your companion's extravagant new bicycle or wishing your accomplice didn't invest such a lot of energy with companions. Help yourself to remember your tough, solid bicycle that gets you where you need to go. Consider the advantages of having an accomplice who likes the worth of fellowship.

In any event, appreciating positive things in your day to day existence that don't identify with envy can assist you with understanding that, while your life may not be awesome (however whose life is?), you've actually got some beneficial things rolling for you.

Practice in-the-moment adapting strategies:

Adapting to jealousy as it comes up will not help you work through hidden causes. Yet, it can assist with keeping the trouble under control until you can manage the basic issues.

Dismissing your consideration from envy can likewise assist with holding you back from following up on your sentiments (and accomplishing something that could hurt a relationship or fellowship).

Do you wind up looking for validation? Asking where your accomplice is going, despite the fact that you know the appropriate response? Harassing them for additional consideration despite the fact that you went through the whole day together? Possibly you over and over get some information about investing energy with a collaborator's companion. These things are an aftereffect of weaknesses in a relationship.

Numerous individuals feel jealous and unreliable in their connections, regardless of whether they are cherished unequivocally by their accomplice. Regardless of whether you're in a generally new relationship or a decades-in length marriage, here's the means by which to quit being uncertain in a relationship.

CAUSES WEAKNESS IN A RELATIONSHIP

In the event that you feel unreliable, this is on the grounds that you haven't managed whatever is placing you in a negative state. This could be that your necessities aren't being met by your relationship, or it could have to do with something outside your association, similar to an absence of fearlessness or dread of the obscure. The significant thing is to get to the base of the issue and settle it together.

1. Start with Confidence

The center reason for weaknesses in a relationship is regularly an absence of self-esteem. In the event that one accomplice clutches unsafe restricting convictions, such as fearing disappointment or imagining that they don't merit love, they will not have the option to trust totally – and trust is the establishment of any relationship. To chip away at confidence, first recognize and beat your restricting convictions. Figure out how to intrude on regrettable examples of self-talk. Find ways to construct your certainty and transform your life into an excursion of revelation, not doubt and doubt.

2. Figure out how to convey adequately

Openness is of the utmost importance in all everyday issues – and that is particularly obvious in case you're feeling unreliable in a relationship. To truly find how to quit being unreliable in a relationship, everything thing you can manage is viably speak with your accomplice. How does your accomplice impart? What's their correspondence style? You can talk things over more than once, however except if you're really interfacing with your accomplice on their level, it will be trying to determine waiting issues.

3. Meet each other's Requirements

Feeling shaky in a relationship is regularly an indication that specific necessities aren't being met. There are six essential human necessities that influence everyone in the world. We as a whole endeavor to feel sure that we can keep away from agony and gain delight; we long for assortment throughout everyday life; we need to feel critical; association with others is fundamental and development and commitment help us discover satisfaction. Every individual positions these requirements in an alternate manner. Which one is generally critical to you? Is your relationship assisting with satisfying this need? If not, how might you work on the relationship to feel more cherished and upheld?

4. Equilibrium your Extremity

Couple managing instability in relationship. In each relationship there is one band together with a manly energy and another with ladylike energy. These energies don't need to line up with sexes, however contradicting powers should be available to discover heartfelt amicability. This idea is called extremity. In case you're feeling uncertain in a relationship, you and your accomplice may not be in balance. On the off chance that the two accomplices take on manly or female qualities, it can make instabilities emerge. Take a gander at how your jobs have changed over the long haul. How might you reestablish extremity and oust frailty?

5. Behave like you are a new couple

At the point when you begin dating another person, the energy is jolting. You need to learn everything about your accomplice and be truly near them at whatever point conceivable. Over the long run, this flash blurs. As you become better familiar with your accomplice, the firecrackers you previously felt begin to fail. You become agreeable in your propensities and quit attempting to intrigue. Frailties in a relationship can surface when your accomplice feels that you're done putting forth an attempt or that your fascination is blurring. Bring back the enthusiasm in your relationship and behave as you did when you began dating. Praise your accomplice. Plan astounding dates. Keep in touch with them love notes. These little demonstrations can reignite the enthusiasm and squash uncertainties.

6. Make new stories

Mix-ups are made in even the most joyful connections, yet feasible connections can leave those missteps before. What are you and your accomplice managing? Regardless of in the event that you've recently battled about accounts or teases, assuming you're choosing to push ahead as a couple, it's an ideal opportunity to abandon those old stories. Rather than demanding that your accomplice consistently accomplishes something that bothers you, take a stab at moving your outlook. Acknowledge your accomplice for what their identity is and choose to make a lovely new story together as opposed to remembering past torment, and you'll figure out how to quit being unreliable in a relationship.

7. Quit over analyzing

The entirety of your instabilities in a relationship start in your own head. Your contemplations influence your feelings, and your feelings influence your activities. At the point when you let restless contemplations winding wild, that is the point at which you lash out at your accomplice, become protective or closed down. Stop these sentiments before they start by figuring out how to control your feelings. Keep your accomplice's activities in context – everybody converses with the other gender, needs to go out with their companions and needs alone time on occasion. This doesn't think about gravely you. It implies you're in a typical, sound relationship!

CHAPTER FOUR

FIXING LOW SELF-ESTEEM IN A RELATIONSHIP

Self-esteem is the assessment you have of yourself. In the event that you have low self-esteem, it can impact your view of yourself and furthermore your close connection. You may not feel deserving of adoration or have extreme feelings of fear of relinquishment. Low confidence can prompt low relationship fulfillment and lower levels of trust and more conflict. Be that as it may, by tweaking the manner in which you connect with your accomplice and by testing your outlook, you can start to roll out certain improvements in your relationship.

1. Tolerating Yourself

Utilize positive affirmations. Focusing on sure self-talk is a decent method to work on your confidence. Attempt to require a couple of moments consistently to say something pleasant to yourself. This can be a basic commendation or essentially advising yourself that you love yourself. Consistently, say (or state), "I cherish and acknowledge myself genuinely for who I'm." For more data, look at How to Work on Confidence with Positive Insistences. Or then again, take a stab at glancing in the mirror and offering yourself a commendation about your actual appearance consistently. For instance, you can say, "I love the way my hair looks today! It is so sparkling and smooth!"

2. Practice self-compassion.

 Acknowledge that you are human and are having a human experience. This can assist you with recollecting that you don't experience alone and that you are associated with others. Everybody commits errors and ends up in circumstances out of their control. Recalling this can assist you with being caring toward yourself as well as other people.

Permit yourself to encounter your feelings. Try not to smother your feelings yet don't detonate, by the same token. Recall that it's entirely expected to have feelings and communicating them is alright. Feelings travel every which way and don't characterize you, regardless of how terrible they feel. For instance, in the event that you feel disregarded by your accomplice, perceive that it's alright to feel awful, yet these feelings don't characterize you or the relationship.

3. Recognize your qualities and weaknesses.

Making a rundown of 10 of your qualities and 10 of your shortcomings is a decent method to begin constructing your confidence. Take a stab at partitioning a piece of paper into two sections and afterward compose 10 of your qualities on one side and 10 of your shortcomings on the other.

Numerous individuals think that it's simple to distinguish shortcomings, however recognizing qualities can be seriously difficult. To recognize your qualities, consider times that individuals have commended you. These can be seemingly insignificant details, for example, times individuals have commented, "You're a decent audience!" or "You are great at drawing!" Regardless of whether you think it does not merit posting, add it to your qualities list.

Make an effort not to contrast yourself with others. All things considered, advise yourself that everybody has something they are acceptable at and center on what you are acceptable at.

4. Put forward practical objectives

 Setting huge, unreasonable objectives can cause a circumstance where you are not living up to your own desires and this can harm your confidence. To keep this from occurring, attempt to lay out sensible objectives for yourself. Ensure that your objectives are explicit and that you have a method of estimating them. For instance, a particular and quantifiable objective may be a like thing, "I need to further develop my mile time by 30 seconds before the month's over."

Assuming your objective is too huge, this can likewise be overpowering. Attempt to break huge objectives into more reasonable ones also. For instance, rather than defining an objective to get a superior line of work, you could lay out more modest objectives for yourself, for example, to chip away at your resume or to go after five new positions each week.

5. Recognize your achievements

 In some cases your achievements may appear to go undetected by individuals, yet you can generally recognize them yourself. Have a go at trying out recognizing the entirety of your achievements, regardless of whether you think they are too little to even consider recognizing.

For instance, in the event that you have been attempting to eat better and you arranged a solid supper for yourself, then, at that point you could take note of this in your diary with something like, "Had steamed broccoli and salmon for supper this evening! Approach to go me!"

Another choice is to glance yourself in the mirror and salute yourself on your achievements. For instance, in the event that you read truly hard for a major test, you may glance yourself in the mirror and say, "You did a great job! I am so pleased with you for all the difficult work you put in!"

6. Take great consideration of yourself

 Taking great consideration of yourself is likewise significant for building confidence. By taking great consideration of your body and brain, you will send the message to yourself that you merit great treatment. A few things you can do to take great consideration of yourself include:

Rehearsing great cleanliness, for example, by showering each day, brushing your hair, brushing your teeth, utilizing antiperspirant, and wearing clean garments.

Making time to do things you appreciate, like playing an instrument, perusing, watching films, or painting.

Dealing with your actual wellbeing, for example, by planning quality dinners for yourself, working out, and getting a lot of rest.

Overseeing pressure, for example, by ruminating, rehearsing yoga, or doing profound breathing activities.

7. See a therapist

In case you're uncertain of where to start or how to see yourself all the more emphatically, treatment can be an incredible spot to begin. Talk treatments like psychological conduct treatment (CBT) can help you start to feel more sure and tolerating of yourself. To discover an advisor, contact your protection supplier, neighborhood emotional wellness center, or get a proposal from a doctor or a companion.

CHAPTER FIVE

INTERACTING WITH YOUR PARTNER

Work on being assertive: Having low confidence may mean you experience issues articulating your thoughts in the relationship. Work on being decisive in your relationship by straightforwardly and sincerely conveying your needs, needs, sentiments, convictions, and opinions. This can help you get comfortable with yourself and permit you to see that your opinion and feel is significant in your relationship.

Don't simply oblige what your accomplice needs to do. For instance, assuming your accomplice needs to see one film and you'd prefer to see an alternate one, shout out and share your desires. Say, "I realize you need an activity film, however I'd like a satire. Is it accurate to say that you are in the mood for seeing two films, or would it be a good idea for us to watch one around evening time and one tomorrow?"

Realize that your requirements are significant. On the off chance that your accomplice is stressed over being late some place, say, "I know you should be on schedule, notwithstanding, I need some an ideal opportunity to eat before we leave."

Accept the positive things your accomplice says about you: In the event that your accomplice discovers you appealing, wise and persevering, acknowledge that these might be characteristics that you possess. While you might rush to overlook or battle these characteristics, you can start to see them in yourself and start to see yourself more like your accomplice sees you over the long run.

On the off chance that you struggle tolerating how your accomplice sees you, ask yourself, "Is it conceivable I may have this quality? When have I seen this quality in myself?"

Try not to continually look for approval: Getting approval from your partner may feel better, yet the impacts are regularly brief and required once more. This can feel like a steady skirmish of needing to have approval and afterward becoming vexed when your partner doesn't offer it to you. Advise yourself that you needn't bother with anybody's approval, either from your folks, companions, and partner. You are advantageous and needn't bother with anybody's endorsement to be adored or thought often about.

 Looking for approval may look like posing inquiries, for example, "Do I glance great in this? Do you cherish me? Am I sufficient for you?"

Try not to depend on praises from your partner to keep up with your confidence. Praises may feel better, yet you may return to negative considerations about yourself or need consistent commendations to have a positive outlook on yourself.

Request help from your partner. Converse with your partner about the particular things you battle with and how you could utilize their help. Request that your accomplice pay attention to you without hindering or attempting to tackle your issues. Request an embrace when you need it. Tell your partner you struggle requesting help, and keeping in mind that you work on communicating your necessities you'd like it on the off chance that they offered help.

Say. "It's difficult for me to request help since I don't feel like I merit it or I would prefer not to trouble you. There are sure things I might want your assistance with and I'd prefer to talk about them with you."

Have some good times together. Do charming things together regularly: Discover a movement that both of you has done previously and go do it together. It tends to be encouraging to have a go at something new realizing that it's new for your accomplice also. In the event that you feel senseless, almost certainly, your accomplice does, as well, and you can giggle about it together. Have a go at swing moving, painting, or attempt another café together.

9 798544 823049